THE HEALING
KITCHEN

EMBRACING WELLNESS, DEFYING CANCER.

Introduction

Are you ready to embark on a culinary journey that defies the odds and empowers your fight against cancer? Look no further than "The Healing Kitchen: Embracing Wellness, Defying Cancer." This groundbreaking cookbook is not just a collection of recipes; it's a powerful tool designed to help you harness the healing potential of food and transform your kitchen into a hub of strength and resilience.

Inside the pages of this book, you'll find a treasure trove of delicious recipes that not only tantalize your taste buds but also work in harmony with your body's natural defenses. Each dish has been thoughtfully crafted, drawing on the latest scientific research and expert knowledge in the field of oncology and nutrition. From nourishing soups to vibrant salads, from hearty mains to delectable desserts, every recipe is a testament to the incredible healing power of food.

But "The Healing Kitchen" goes beyond just recipes. It's a comprehensive guide that empowers you to make informed choices about the foods you eat and the impact they can have on your journey to wellness. Packed with evidence-based information, practical tips, and insightful guidance, this book equips you with the knowledge and tools needed to take charge of your health.

Discover how to incorporate cancer-fighting ingredients into your everyday meals, learn about the benefits of specific nutrients, and explore innovative cooking techniques that maximize the bioavailability of nutrients. With "The Healing Kitchen," you'll not only nourish your body but also nurture your spirit, finding solace and strength in the act of preparing wholesome meals for yourself and your loved ones.

Prepare to be inspired as you read empowering stories of individuals who have defied the odds and triumphed over cancer, sharing their personal experiences and the role that nutrition played in their healing journeys. Their stories serve as a reminder that you are not alone in this fight and that there is hope and resilience to be found within the walls of your kitchen.

"The Healing Kitchen: Embracing Wellness, Defying Cancer" is not just a cookbook; it's a lifeline—a beacon of hope that encourages you to take an active role in your own healing. So, tie on your apron, grab your spatula, and let the power of food guide you on a remarkable path toward wellness and victory over cancer.

TABLE OF CONTENTS

CHAPTER ONE

Introduction: Embracing Wellness through Food

Section 1.1: Setting the Stage
In this opening section, we will set the stage for the profound impact that nutrition can have on cancer prevention and treatment. We'll explore the growing body of scientific evidence that demonstrates the connection between food and healing, highlighting how the right choices in the kitchen can become powerful allies in your fight against cancer. By emphasizing the importance of nutrition as a holistic approach to wellness, we will lay the foundation for the transformative journey that awaits you in "The Healing Kitchen."

Section 1. 2: The Link between Food and Healing
Here, we will delve deeper into the intricate link between food and healing. Drawing upon scientific research and expert insights, we will explore how certain nutrients, antioxidants, and phytochemicals found in various foods can play a crucial role in preventing and combating cancer. We will demystify the complex mechanisms through which these compounds work, shedding light on their ability to fight inflammation, oxidative stress, and the growth of cancer cells. By understanding the science behind the healing power of food, you will

be empowered to make informed choices in your kitchen.

Section 1. 3: Empowering Your Health Journey
In this section, we will empower you to take an active role in your health journey by embracing wellness through food. We will discuss the importance of adopting a positive mindset and cultivating a sense of empowerment when it comes to your dietary choices. By recognizing that you have the ability to nourish and support your body's natural defenses, you can shift from a passive role to an active one, making intentional decisions in the kitchen that align with your goals and aspirations.

Section 1.4: The Power of Personalization
Every individual's cancer journey is unique, and their nutritional needs may vary. In this section, we will emphasize the significance of personalized nutrition and highlight the importance of working with healthcare professionals, such as registered dietitians or oncology nutritionists, to develop a tailored approach that suits your specific circumstances. We will provide guidance on how to navigate the vast amount of information available and help you discern evidence-based recommendations from unfounded claims.

Section1. 5: Navigating the Chapters Ahead
To provide a glimpse of the exciting content that awaits you in "The Healing Kitchen," we will provide

an overview of the chapters and sections to come. We will touch upon the diverse range of recipes, nutrition insights, and practical tips that will equip you to transform your kitchen into a hub of strength and resilience. By offering this roadmap, we aim to ignite your curiosity and anticipation for the empowering information and delicious recipes that lie ahead.

In conclusion, this opening chapter has laid the groundwork for your journey through "The Healing Kitchen." By emphasizing the powerful connection between food and wellness, we have set the stage for a transformative experience. Armed with knowledge and understanding, you are ready to embrace the role of nutrition in your fight against cancer. With each turn of the page, you will discover the healing potential of the ingredients in your pantry, the science behind their effects, and the practical strategies to incorporate them into your daily life. So, let us embark on this culinary voyage together, and may "The Healing Kitchen" become your beacon of hope and empowerment on the path to wellness.

CHAPTER TWO
The Science of Cancer-Fighting Foods

Section 2.1: Nutrients: The Building Blocks of Health

In this section, we will explore the vital role that nutrients play in cancer prevention and treatment. We will delve into the specific nutrients, such as vitamins, minerals, and phytonutrients, that have been shown to have powerful anti-cancer properties. By understanding the functions and sources of these nutrients, you will be equipped with the knowledge to make informed choices about the foods you consume.

Section 2.2: Antioxidants: Neutralizing Free Radicals

Free radicals, unstable molecules that can damage cells and contribute to the development of cancer, are a constant presence in our bodies. However, antioxidants found in certain foods have the ability to neutralize these harmful molecules. We will discuss the importance of incorporating antioxidant-rich foods into your diet, such as berries, leafy greens, and nuts, and how they can help protect against oxidative stress and support overall health.

Section 2.3: Phytochemicals: Nature's Cancer-Fighting Compounds

Phytochemicals are natural compounds found in plant-based foods that have been shown to have powerful anti-cancer effects. We will explore the diverse range of phytochemicals, such as carotenoids, flavonoids, and polyphenols, and their potential mechanisms of action against cancer cells. By highlighting specific food sources that are rich in these compounds, we will empower you to incorporate them into your meals and snacks.

Section 2.4: Fiber: Nourishing the Gut Microbiome

The health of our gut microbiome, the community of microorganisms in our digestive tract, has a profound impact on our overall well-being, including our risk of developing cancer. Dietary fiber plays a crucial role in supporting a diverse and healthy gut microbiome. We will discuss the importance of consuming fiber-rich foods, such as whole grains, legumes, and fruits, and how they can contribute to a balanced and thriving gut ecosystem.

Section 2.5: Beyond Nutrients: Whole Foods and Synergy

While individual nutrients and compounds are important, it is essential to emphasize the power of whole foods and the synergistic effects of their components. We will discuss the benefits of consuming a varied and balanced diet that includes a wide range of whole foods. By embracing the concept of food synergy, where the combination of different nutrients and compounds in whole foods creates greater health benefits than isolated nutrients, you can optimize the potential anti-cancer effects of your meals.

Section 2.6: Mindful Eating for Cancer Prevention and Recovery

In this section, we will explore the concept of mindful eating and its relevance to cancer prevention and recovery. By cultivating a mindful approach to eating, you can foster a deeper connection with your body, enhance your enjoyment of meals, and make conscious choices that support your health goals. We will provide practical tips and techniques for incorporating mindfulness into your eating habits, allowing you to savor each bite and nourish your body and mind.

This chapter has delved into the science behind cancer-fighting foods, highlighting the essential nutrients, antioxidants, phytochemicals, and fiber that contribute to their powerful effects. By understanding the role of these components, as well as the importance of whole foods and mindful eating, you are now equipped with the knowledge to make informed dietary choices that support your journey to wellness. In the chapters ahead, we will explore how to translate this knowledge into practical, delicious recipes that harness the healing power of food in the Beat Cancer Kitchen.

CHAPTER THREE
building a Cancer-Fighting Pantry

Section 3.1: Stocking the Essentials
In this section, we will guide you through the process of building a cancer-fighting pantry. We will identify the essential ingredients that form the foundation of a well-stocked kitchen focused on promoting health and wellness. From whole grains and legumes to spices and herbs, we will discuss the nutritional benefits of each item and provide tips on sourcing and storing them for maximum freshness and potency.

Section 3.2: Whole Foods, Fresh Flavors
Incorporating whole foods into your diet is key to supporting your body's natural defenses against cancer. We will explore the benefits of choosing whole, unprocessed foods and discuss how to identify them at the grocery store. By opting for fresh produce, whole grains, and minimally processed ingredients, you can enhance the nutritional value of your meals and savor the vibrant flavors that nature provides.

Section 3.3: Herbs and Spices: The Healing Kitchen's Secret Weapons
Herbs and spices not only add depth and complexity to your dishes but also offer an array of health benefits .We will explore the medicinal properties of various herbs and spices, such as

turmeric, ginger, garlic, and rosemary, that have been shown to possess potent anti-cancer properties. We will provide guidance on how to select, store, and use these flavorful additions to elevate the nutritional value of your meals while enhancing taste and aroma.

Section 3.4: Embracing Good Fats
Contrary to popular belief, not all fats are detrimental to your health. In fact, certain fats can be beneficial and support your body's anti-cancer defenses. We will discuss the importance of incorporating healthy fats, such as avocado, nuts, seeds, and olive oil, into your cooking. By understanding the role of these fats in promoting optimal cellular function and reducing inflammation, you can make conscious choices that support your well-being.

Section 3.5: Minimizing Harmful Additives and Chemicals
A cancer-fighting pantry is not just about what you include but also what you exclude. We will discuss the importance of reading labels and avoiding harmful additives, preservatives, and artificial ingredients. By opting for organic produce, minimizing processed foods, and choosing natural sweeteners, you can reduce your exposure to potentially harmful chemicals and create a safer, cleaner kitchen environment.

Section 3.6: Meal Planning and Batch Cooking
Efficient meal planning and batch cooking are essential strategies for maintaining a cancer-fighting kitchen. We will provide practical tips and techniques for effective meal planning, including recipe selection, ingredient prep, and storage. By incorporating these strategies into your routine, you can save time, reduce stress, and ensure that your meals are balanced, nutritious, and ready to enjoy even on busy days.

This chapter has focused on building a cancer-fighting pantry, providing guidance on stocking essential ingredients, embracing whole foods, harnessing the power of herbs and spices, incorporating healthy fats, and minimizing harmful additives. By curating a pantry that supports your health goals, you can create a solid foundation for preparing nourishing meals in the Beat Cancer Kitchen. In the chapters ahead, we will dive into the delicious recipes that will transform these pantry staples into vibrant and healing dishes, empowering you to take charge of your well-being one ingredient at a time.

CHAPTER FOUR
Nutrient-Packed Starters and Nourishing Soups

Section 4.1: Appetizers for Health and Flavor
In this section, we will explore nutrient-packed starters that not only tantalize your taste buds but also provide a powerful dose of cancer-fighting nutrients. From colorful vegetable crudités with flavorful dips to homemade hummus variations, we will showcase appetizer recipes that are rich in antioxidants, fiber, and essential vitamins and minerals. These vibrant and delicious starters will set the tone for a nourishing meal while supporting your overall health and well-being.

Section 4.2: Nourishing Soups for Healing and Comfort
Soups have long been known for their comforting and healing properties. In this section, we will delve into the world of nourishing soups that are designed to support your body's immune system and promote overall wellness. From hearty vegetable soups to broths infused with immune-boosting herbs and spices, we will provide recipes that not only warm your soul but also provide essential nutrients for your body's healing journey.

Section 4.3: Superfoods in Every Spoonful
Superfoods are nutrient powerhouses that offer an abundance of health benefits. We will highlight the inclusion of superfoods in both starters and soups,

discussing their specific properties that make them particularly beneficial in fighting cancer. Whether it's adding leafy greens like kale and spinach, incorporating antioxidant-rich berries, or utilizing healing herbs like turmeric and ginger, we will guide you in creating recipes that showcase the nutritional prowess of these superfoods.

Section 4.4: Comforting Bowls of Nourishment
Bowls have become a popular trend for their versatility, simplicity, and nutritional balance. We will explore nourishing bowl recipes that incorporate a variety of cancer-fighting ingredients, such as whole grains, lean proteins, and an abundance of colorful vegetables. These balanced and satisfying bowls will provide a convenient and delicious way to pack your meals with essential nutrients while offering endless options for customization and creativity.

Section 4.5: Tailoring Starters and Soups to Dietary Needs
In this section, we will address various dietary needs and restrictions, providing tips and substitutions to accommodate different eating preferences. Whether you follow a plant-based diet, have specific food allergies or intolerances, or require modifications based on your treatment plan, we will offer guidance on adapting the recipes to suit your individual needs. Empowering you with options and alternatives, we aim to ensure that

everyone can enjoy the nourishing and flavorful starters and soups in the Beat Cancer Kitchen.

Section 4.6: Preparation Tips and Make-Ahead Options

Preparing starters and soups can be made easier and more convenient with the right techniques and planning. We will share practical tips for efficient ingredient preparation, time-saving cooking methods, and make-ahead options that allow you to enjoy these nutrient-packed dishes even on busy days. By incorporating these strategies into your routine, you can seamlessly incorporate starters and soups into your cancer-fighting meal plan without compromising on flavor or nutrition.

This chapter has introduced you to a world of nutrient-packed starters and nourishing soups that contribute to your overall health and well-being. By incorporating antioxidant-rich ingredients, superfoods, and comforting flavors, these recipes provide a delightful and nourishing start to your meals. We have also addressed various dietary needs and offered preparation tips to ensure that these dishes can be enjoyed by all. In the chapters ahead, we will continue to explore the delicious recipes that await you in the Beat Cancer Kitchen, helping you make every spoonful a step towards optimal health and healing.

CHAPTER FIVE
Wholesome Main Courses for Sustained Strength

Section 5.1: Plant-Powered Plates
In this section, we will celebrate the abundance of plant-based ingredients that can form the foundation of wholesome main courses. From hearty grain bowls and protein-rich legume dishes to creative vegetable-based entrées, we will showcase recipes that showcase the versatility and nutrient density of plant-powered plates. These dishes will provide sustained strength and nourishment while offering a delicious and satisfying dining experience.

Section 5.2: Lean Proteins and Seafood Delights
While plant-based options are valuable, lean proteins and seafood can also play a role in supporting your nutritional needs. We will explore recipes that feature lean protein sources, such as poultry, fish, and tofu, which provide essential amino acids and micronutrients. Additionally, we will highlight the health benefits of incorporating seafood rich in omega-3 fatty acids, such as salmon and sardines, into your diet for their anti-inflammatory properties and potential cancer-fighting effects.

Section 5.3: Wholesome Grains and Smart Carbohydrates

Whole grains and smart carbohydrates are vital sources of energy and essential nutrients. In this section, we will showcase recipes that embrace wholesome grains like quinoa, brown rice, and whole wheat pasta as the base for nourishing main courses. We will also explore the benefits of smart carbohydrates, such as sweet potatoes, lentils, and beans, which provide a slow release of energy and contribute to a balanced meal that supports your overall health and well-being.

Section 5.4: Creative Vegetable Medleys
Vegetables are not merely side dishes but can take center stage in a flavorful and nutrient-packed main course. We will inspire you with creative vegetable medleys and plant-based recipes that highlight the vibrant colors, textures, and flavors of seasonal produce. From roasted vegetable tarts and stuffed bell peppers to cauliflower steaks and zucchini noodles, we will demonstrate the versatility and culinary potential of vegetables in creating wholesome and satisfying meals.

Section 5.5: Sauces, Dressings, and Flavor Enhancers
A well-prepared sauce or dressing can elevate a simple dish to a culinary masterpiece. In this section, we will explore the art of creating flavorful and nutrient-rich sauces, dressings, and flavor enhancers that complement your main courses. We will discuss the use of herbs, spices, and natural

ingredients to add depth and complexity to your dishes while maximizing their nutritional benefits. With these versatile additions, you can enhance the flavor profile of your meals without compromising on health.

Section 5.6: Adapting Main Courses for Dietary Preferences
Individual dietary preferences and restrictions should not limit your culinary experience. In this section, we will provide guidance on adapting main course recipes to accommodate various dietary needs, such as vegetarian, vegan, gluten-free, and dairy-free diets. We will offer ingredient substitutions and preparation tips to ensure that everyone can enjoy the wholesome and flavorful main courses in the Beat Cancer Kitchen, regardless of their individual requirements.

This chapter has explored the realm of wholesome main courses that provide sustained strength and nourishment. From plant-powered plates and lean proteins to creative vegetable medleys and flavorful sauces, these recipes offer a wide array of options to suit different tastes and dietary preferences. By incorporating nutrient-dense ingredients and highlighting the culinary potential of each component, we have presented a variety of dishes that will make your mealtimes satisfying and enjoyable while promoting your overall health and well-being. As we venture into the following chapters, we will continue to unravel the delicious recipes and transformative power of the Beat Cancer Kitchen.

CHAPTER SIX
Wholesome Sides and Vibrant Salads

Section 6.1: Sides That Steal the Show
In this section, we will showcase wholesome sides that are not mere accompaniments but steal the show with their flavor and nutritional value. From roasted seasonal vegetables and vibrant grain salads to creative twists on classic side dishes, we will provide recipes that elevate your meal and contribute to your overall health. These sides will add color, texture, and a delightful array of flavors to your plate, making every bite a celebration of wholesome eating.

Section 6.2: Powerhouse Salads
Salads can be so much more than a simple mix of greens. In this section, we will explore powerhouse salads that incorporate an abundance of nutrient-rich ingredients. From colorful fruit and vegetable combinations to grain-based salads packed with protein and fiber, we will provide recipes that showcase the beauty and versatility of salads. These vibrant creations will not only nourish your body but also please your palate with a variety of tastes and textures.

Section 6.3: Dressings and Vinaigrettes for Flavorful Greens
The right dressing can transform a basic salad into a culinary delight. We will delve into the world of

homemade dressings and vinaigrettes, exploring a range of flavors and highlighting the use of fresh herbs, tangy citrus, and healthy fats. Whether you prefer creamy dressings or light and zesty vinaigrettes, we will provide recipes that will enhance the flavors of your greens and make your salads irresistible.

Section 6.4: Embracing Seasonal Produce
Seasonal produce offers the freshest and most flavorful ingredients. In this section, we will emphasize the importance of embracing seasonal fruits and vegetables in your sides and salads. We will discuss the benefits of eating locally and highlight the nutritional advantages of consuming produce at its peak. By incorporating seasonal ingredients, you can savor the vibrant flavors and maximize the nutrient content of your dishes.

Section 6.5: Balanced Sides and Salads for Every Meal
Wholesome sides and salads can enhance any meal, from breakfast to dinner. We will provide ideas and recipes for incorporating these dishes into your daily routine, ensuring a balanced and nutritious eating experience throughout the day. Whether you're seeking a refreshing salad for lunch, a hearty side for dinner, or a creative twist for brunch, we will inspire you with options that align with your mealtime preferences.

Section 6.6: Preparing Ahead and Storage Tips
Efficient meal planning and preparation can make incorporating sides and salads into your routine seamless. We will share practical tips for prepping ingredients ahead of time, storing salads for maximum freshness, and repurposing leftovers to minimize food waste. These strategies will help you save time and ensure that you always have nourishing sides and salads readily available to complement your meals.

This chapter has explored the realm of wholesome sides and vibrant salads, showcasing their potential to steal the show and contribute to your overall health. From creative and flavorful sides to nutrient-packed salads, we have provided recipes that celebrate the beauty of seasonal produce and elevate your meals with an array of tastes and textures. By embracing these recipes and incorporating them into your daily routine, you can make every meal a delicious and nutritious experience in the Beat Cancer Kitchen. As we continue our journey through the following chapters, we will uncover more delightful recipes and insights to empower you on your path to optimal health and wellness.

CHAPTER SEVEN
Sweet and Wholesome Desserts

Section 7.1: Redefining Desserts with Nutritious Ingredients

In this section, we will redefine the concept of desserts by incorporating wholesome and nutritious ingredients. We will explore how you can satisfy your sweet tooth while nourishing your body with recipes that utilize natural sweeteners, whole grains, and antioxidant-rich ingredients. From fruit-based treats to innovative twists on classic desserts, we will showcase how desserts can be a delightful and guilt-free part of your cancer-fighting journey.

Section 7.2: Fruits and Berries: Nature's Sweet Delights

Fruits and berries not only offer natural sweetness but are also packed with essential vitamins, minerals, and antioxidants. We will highlight the nutritional benefits of various fruits and berries and provide recipes that showcase their flavors and health-promoting properties. From refreshing fruit salads to baked fruit desserts, these recipes will allow you to indulge in the goodness of nature while satisfying your dessert cravings.

Section 7.3: Whole Grains and Healthy Treats

Whole grains offer a nutritious alternative to refined flours and can be incorporated into desserts for added fiber and essential nutrients. We will explore recipes that feature whole grains such as oats, quinoa, and whole wheat flour, creating treats that are both wholesome and delicious. From hearty muffins to homemade granola bars, these desserts will provide sustained energy and satisfy your sweet tooth without compromising on nutrition.

Section 7.4: Creative Treats with Nuts and Seeds
Nuts and seeds are not only a great source of healthy fats but also contribute a delightful crunch and depth of flavor to desserts. We will showcase recipes that incorporate a variety of nuts and seeds, such as almonds, walnuts, chia seeds, and flaxseeds. From energy balls and nut butter-based treats to seed crackers and homemade granola, these desserts will provide a satisfying and nutrient-dense indulgence.

Section 7.5: Lightened-Up Versions of Classic Desserts
In this section, we will explore lightened-up versions of classic desserts, offering healthier alternatives without compromising on taste. We will provide recipes that utilize smart substitutions, such as reducing sugar, incorporating alternative flours, and utilizing healthier fats. From guilt-free chocolate mousse to nutrient-rich fruit crumbles, these desserts will allow you to enjoy your favorites while nourishing your body.

Section 7.6: Desserts for Special Occasions
Special occasions call for special desserts. In this
section, we will present recipes for celebratory
treats that are both indulgent and nutritious.
Whether you're planning a birthday party or a
holiday gathering, we will provide recipes for cakes,
pies, and other festive desserts that prioritize
wholesome ingredients and maximize flavor. These
desserts will allow you to savor the joy of special
occasions while staying true to your health goals.

This chapter has reimagined desserts as sweet and
wholesome treats that can be enjoyed as part of
your cancer-fighting journey. By utilizing nutritious
ingredients, such as fruits, whole grains, nuts, and
seeds, we have showcased recipes that satisfy
your cravings while nourishing your body. Whether
it's indulging in fruity delights, exploring whole grain
treats, or enjoying lightened-up versions of classics,
these desserts offer a delicious and guilt-free way
to end your meals in the Beat Cancer Kitchen. As
we venture into the following chapters, we will
continue to uncover delightful recipes and insights
that support your overall health and well-being.

CHAPTER EIGHT
Mindful Eating and Wellness Practices

Section 8.1: The Power of Mindful Eating
In this section, we will delve into the concept of mindful eating and its profound impact on our overall well-being. We will explore the benefits of slowing down, savoring each bite, and paying attention to our body's hunger and fullness cues. By incorporating mindful eating practices into our daily lives, we can enhance our relationship with food, promote better digestion, and cultivate a deeper sense of gratitude and enjoyment during mealtime.

Section 8.2: Nourishing the Mind-Body Connection
The mind-body connection plays a crucial role in our overall health and wellness. In this section, we will discuss how our thoughts, emotions, and stress levels can influence our eating habits and digestion. We will explore techniques such as meditation, deep breathing exercises, and mindful movement to cultivate a sense of calm and balance. By nourishing the mind-body connection, we can create a supportive environment for healing and well-being.

Section 8.3: Building Healthy Habits
Creating sustainable and healthy habits is essential for long-term well-being. We will provide guidance on how to build healthy eating habits that align with

your cancer-fighting goals. From meal planning and mindful grocery shopping to practical tips for portion control and mindful snacking, we will empower you with strategies that make healthy choices a natural part of your lifestyle.

Section 8.4: Finding Joy in Movement
Physical activity is a vital component of a healthy lifestyle. We will discuss the importance of finding joy in movement and incorporating enjoyable activities into your daily routine. Whether it's yoga, walking, dancing, or any other form of exercise that resonates with you, we will explore how movement can improve your mood, boost your energy levels, and support your overall well-being.

Section 8.5: Cultivating Self-Care and Stress Management
Self-care and stress management are integral to maintaining a balanced and healthy lifestyle. We will discuss the importance of self-care practices such as adequate sleep, relaxation techniques, and engaging in activities that bring you joy and peace. Additionally, we will explore stress management strategies to help you navigate the challenges that may arise during your cancer-fighting journey.

Section 8.6: Creating a Supportive Environment
The environment in which we eat and live has a significant impact on our well-being. We will provide tips on creating a supportive environment that

fosters healthy habits and promotes mindful eating. From organizing your kitchen for success to cultivating a positive and nurturing atmosphere at the dining table, we will guide you in creating an environment that supports your overall wellness.

This chapter has explored the importance of mindful eating and wellness practices in our cancer-fighting journey. By embracing mindful eating, nurturing the mind-body connection, and cultivating healthy habits, we can create a foundation of well-being that extends beyond our meals. Incorporating joyful movement, self-care, and stress management techniques further enhances our overall health and resilience. As we conclude this chapter, we encourage you to integrate these practices into your daily life, creating a supportive environment that nourishes both your body and mind in the Beat Cancer Kitchen. In the chapters ahead, we will continue to unravel the transformative power of mindful eating and holistic wellness, empowering you on your path to optimal health and healing.

CHAPTER NINE
Nurturing Connections and Support

Section 9.1: The Importance of Community
In this section, we will emphasize the significance of nurturing connections and seeking support during your cancer-fighting journey. We will explore the role of community in providing encouragement, empathy, and a sense of belonging. From support groups to online forums and local resources, we will guide you in finding and fostering a supportive network that understands and embraces your unique challenges and triumphs.

Section 9.2: Cultivating Relationships in the Beat Cancer Kitchen
The kitchen can serve as a space for nurturing relationships and fostering connection. We will discuss the joy of cooking and sharing meals with loved ones and explore ways to involve family and friends in the culinary experience. From collaborative meal planning to cooking together and hosting gatherings, we will provide ideas and strategies for creating meaningful connections through food and the Beat Cancer Kitchen.

Section 9.3: Communicating Your Needs and Boundaries

Effective communication is crucial when navigating the challenges of a cancer journey. In this section, we will explore strategies for expressing your needs, setting boundaries, and seeking support from your loved ones and healthcare team. We will discuss open and honest communication, active listening, and the importance of self-advocacy in ensuring that your needs are met throughout your healing process.

Section 9.4: Integrating Mind-Body Therapies
Mind-body therapies offer additional avenues for support and healing. We will explore practices such as meditation, yoga, acupuncture, and massage therapy, which can complement conventional treatments and enhance overall well-being. These therapies promote relaxation, reduce stress, and foster a sense of connection between the mind, body, and spirit.

Section 9.5: Celebrating Milestones and Victories
It's important to acknowledge and celebrate milestones and victories, no matter how small, during your cancer-fighting journey. In this section, we will discuss the importance of recognizing and honoring your progress and achievements. We will provide ideas for celebrating milestones, such as completing treatments, reaching wellness goals, and embracing moments of joy, and how to incorporate them into your healing journey.

Section 9.6: Giving Back and Supporting Others Supporting others who are going through similar experiences can be a source of strength and purpose. We will explore ways to give back to the cancer community and support others on their healing journeys. Whether it's through volunteering, sharing your story, or participating in advocacy initiatives, we will inspire you to make a positive impact and foster a sense of connection and solidarity.

This chapter has highlighted the importance of nurturing connections and seeking support throughout your cancer-fighting journey. By cultivating relationships, communicating your needs, integrating mind-body therapies, and celebrating milestones, you can create a supportive and uplifting environment that enhances your healing process. Additionally, giving back to the cancer community allows you to find purpose and strength in supporting others. As we conclude this chapter, we encourage you to embrace the power of connections and support in the Beat Cancer Kitchen and beyond. In the remaining chapters, we will continue to provide insights and resources that empower you to thrive and find solace in the company of others on this transformative journey.

CHAPTER TEN
Long-Term Wellness and Lifestyle Strategies

Section 10.1: Embracing a Lifelong Commitment to Health

In this section, we will discuss the importance of embracing a lifelong commitment to health and wellness beyond the cancer-fighting journey. We will explore the concept of survivorship and how to navigate life after cancer, focusing on long-term wellness strategies that promote overall well-being. From maintaining healthy habits to ongoing self-care and monitoring, we will provide guidance on cultivating a sustainable and thriving lifestyle.

Section 10.2: Continual Nutrition Education and Exploration

Nutrition is a dynamic field, and there is always more to learn and explore. In this section, we will emphasize the importance of continued nutrition education and staying informed about the latest research and developments. We will provide resources and strategies for staying up-to-date with nutritional information, empowering you to make informed choices and adapt your diet as new knowledge emerges.

Section 10.3: Regular Screening and Follow-Up Care

Regular screening and follow-up care are essential components of long-term wellness. We will discuss the importance of staying vigilant with routine check-ups, cancer screenings, and follow-up appointments. By prioritizing proactive healthcare, you can detect any potential issues early on and ensure that you are receiving the necessary support and guidance for maintaining your well-being.

Section 10.4: Mindful Stress Management for Resilience

Stress management is an ongoing practice that supports overall wellness. We will explore various mindful stress management techniques, such as meditation, journaling, and relaxation exercises, that can help build resilience and promote emotional well-being. By incorporating these strategies into your daily life, you can effectively manage stress and cultivate a sense of balance and calm.

Section 10.5: Adapting to Changing Needs and Goals

As time goes on, your needs and goals may evolve. In this section, we will discuss the importance of adapting to these changes and finding flexibility in your wellness journey. We will provide insights on reassessing your nutrition and lifestyle choices, adjusting your exercise routine, and seeking support as you navigate new phases of your life.

Section 10.6: Celebrating Life and Finding Meaning
The final section of this chapter focuses on celebrating life and finding meaning beyond cancer. We will explore the power of gratitude, cultivating positive emotions, and engaging in activities that bring joy and fulfillment. By embracing a mindset of celebration and finding purpose in your life, you can create a fulfilling and meaningful post-cancer existence.

This chapter marks the culmination of your journey in the Beat Cancer Kitchen, as we explore long-term wellness and lifestyle strategies. By embracing a lifelong commitment to health, continuing to educate yourself, prioritizing regular screening and follow-up care, practicing mindful stress management, adapting to changing needs, and finding meaning in life, you can create a sustainable and fulfilling post-cancer lifestyle. As we conclude this chapter and the book as a whole, we celebrate your resilience, strength, and dedication to your well-being. May the knowledge and insights gained from the Beat Cancer Kitchen guide you on a path of lasting health, happiness, and thriving. Remember, you have the power to shape your future and embrace a life filled with vitality and purpose.

CHAPTER ELEVEN
Beyond the Kitchen: Holistic Wellness in Daily Life

Section 11.1: Creating a Healthy Home Environment

In this section, we will explore the importance of creating a healthy home environment that supports your overall well-being. We will discuss strategies for reducing exposure to toxins, improving indoor air quality, and creating a calming and nurturing space. From choosing natural cleaning products to incorporating houseplants and enhancing natural lighting, we will guide you in transforming your home into a sanctuary of health and wellness.

Section 11.2: Mindful Movement and Exercise
Physical activity goes beyond the kitchen and plays
a vital role in holistic wellness. We will delve deeper
into mindful movement and its benefits for the body,
mind, and spirit. From exploring different types of
exercise to incorporating movement into your daily
routine, we will provide insights and practical tips
for finding joy in physical activity and reaping its
numerous rewards.

Section 11.3: Enhancing Sleep Quality
Quality sleep is a cornerstone of well-being. In this
section, we will discuss the importance of sleep and
strategies for improving sleep quality. We will
explore healthy sleep habits, creating a
sleep-friendly environment, and relaxation
techniques that promote restful sleep. By
prioritizing sleep, you can enhance your body's
natural healing processes and support overall
vitality.

Section 11.4: Cultivating a Mindful and Balanced
Lifestyle
Mindfulness and balance are key pillars of holistic
wellness. We will explore practices such as
meditation, mindfulness exercises, and stress
reduction techniques that can help you cultivate a
more present and balanced lifestyle. By embracing
these practices, you can enhance self-awareness,

reduce stress, and foster a sense of peace and contentment in your daily life.

Section 11.5: Nurturing Relationships and Connection
Human connection and nurturing relationships are essential for our overall well-being. We will discuss the significance of fostering healthy relationships, setting boundaries, and engaging in meaningful social interactions. From practicing active listening to expressing gratitude and kindness, we will explore strategies for deepening connections and experiencing the transformative power of positive relationships.

Section 11.6: Embracing the Joy of Nature
Nature has a profound impact on our well-being. In this section, we will emphasize the importance of connecting with nature and incorporating outdoor activities into your daily life. From walking in nature to gardening and outdoor mindfulness practices, we will explore how immersing yourself in the natural world can rejuvenate your spirit, reduce stress, and enhance your overall sense of well-being.

This chapter invites you to expand your journey beyond the kitchen and embrace holistic wellness in your daily life. By creating a healthy home environment, engaging in mindful movement, prioritizing quality sleep, cultivating mindfulness and balance, nurturing relationships, and connecting with nature, you can experience a profound transformation in your overall well-being. As we conclude this chapter and reach the end of the book, we celebrate your commitment to holistic wellness and the strides you have made on your cancer-fighting journey. May the knowledge and practices shared in the Beat Cancer Kitchen continue to guide you towards a life of vibrant health, balance, and fulfillment. Remember, the power to live a holistic and thriving life lies within you.

CHAPTER TWELVE
Sustaining Your Beat Cancer Lifestyle

Section 12.1: The Importance of Sustainability
In this section, we will discuss the significance of sustainability in maintaining your Beat Cancer lifestyle. We will explore the long-term benefits of sustainable choices and practices, both for your own well-being and the well-being of the planet.

From conscious consumption to eco-friendly habits, we will provide insights and strategies for integrating sustainability into your everyday life.

Section 12.2: Mindful Food Choices
Mindful food choices are vital in sustaining your Beat Cancer lifestyle. We will delve deeper into the importance of selecting nutrient-dense foods, incorporating a variety of fruits and vegetables, and making conscious decisions about the sources and production methods of your food. We will explore strategies for ethical eating, supporting local farmers, and reducing food waste, enabling you to nourish your body while contributing to a more sustainable food system.

Section 12.3: Continued Education and Growth
Continued education and personal growth are key to sustaining your Beat Cancer lifestyle. In this section, we will discuss the importance of staying informed about advancements in nutrition, wellness, and cancer research. We will provide resources and strategies for ongoing learning, such as attending seminars, reading reputable publications, and engaging with health professionals, empowering you to continually evolve and enhance your understanding of optimal health practices.

Section 12.4: Building Resilience and Managing Setbacks

Sustaining your Beat Cancer lifestyle requires resilience and the ability to manage setbacks effectively. We will explore techniques for building emotional resilience, navigating challenges, and maintaining a positive mindset. From practicing self-compassion to developing coping strategies, we will equip you with the tools necessary to overcome obstacles and stay committed to your long-term well-being.

Section 12.5: Embracing Flexibility and Adaptability

Flexibility and adaptability are essential in sustaining your Beat Cancer lifestyle. We will discuss the importance of embracing change, adjusting your approach when needed, and finding a balance between structure and flexibility. By cultivating adaptability, you can navigate different life circumstances and maintain your commitment to health and wellness.

Section 12.6: Sharing Your Journey and Inspiring Others

Sharing your Beat Cancer journey and inspiring others can be a powerful way to sustain your lifestyle. We will explore the importance of sharing your experiences, insights, and knowledge with your community and beyond. From blogging and social media to support groups and public speaking, we will discuss ways to use your story to uplift others and create a positive ripple effect in the world.

This chapter emphasizes the sustainability of your Beat Cancer lifestyle. By embracing sustainable practices, making mindful food choices, continuing your education, building resilience, and adapting to change, you can ensure the long-term success and impact of your journey. Remember, sustaining your lifestyle is not just about personal well-being; it is also about making a positive contribution to the planet and inspiring others along the way. As we conclude this chapter and the book, we celebrate your commitment to sustaining your Beat Cancer lifestyle and the transformative effects it has had on your life. May your journey continue to inspire and uplift others, and may you find joy and fulfillment in living a sustainable, vibrant, and thriving life.

www.ingramcontent.com/pod-product-compliance
Lightning Source LLC
Chambersburg PA
CBHW071007260726
48661CB00007B/2832